A Finger Up Your ….

by
Doug Gray

A Finger Up Your....

First published 2009

Published by

Love Your Prostate
Lower Mead
East Camps Bay
Downderry
Cornwall
PL11 3LQ

In the interest of providing greater public awareness of the symptoms and risks of prostate cancer and the need for men to take control of their own screening programme any part of this book may be copied and circulated to meet these objectives.

Also, member organisations of the Prostate Cancer Support Federation are permitted to have an account with the printer below to purchase at cost and distribute copies as required to meet their own awareness and donation income needs, providing prior permission is obtained from the publisher.

Printed by:

Think*Ink*
11-13 Philip Road
Ipswich
Suffolk
IP2 8BH
England

ISBN: 978-0-9563559-0-4
Copyright © Doug Gray

Disclaimer

Although the Author has made his best endeavours to provide factual and accurate information, as well as sound opinions and logical conclusions based on a number of reliable information sources, there is the possibility of errors. For these reasons, the Author cannot accept any liability as a consequence of the information provided in this book.

Dedication

This book is dedicated to my wife Janice for her understanding, care and support during my selfish act of writing this book and leading a campaign for the greater public awareness of the symptoms and risks of prostate cancer.

This book is also dedicated to the thousands of men that have already died and will continue to die unnecessarily of prostate cancer. This is because of the UK Department of Health's decision not to implement national screening and not to provide greater public awareness of the disease.

A Letter from the Author

7th September 2009

Dear Reader,

You might be asking yourself why I have written this book when I am not an expert on prostate cancer or a health professional?

The answer is simple. I was ignorant of the early warning signs. I also believed that prostate cancer was a disease that only affected old men. Also, I didn't class myself as old when I experienced the first signs at just turned 61 years of age.

When diagnosed, after an emergency admission into hospital in late January 2009 at the age of 62, a hospital doctor said that my life expectancy could be as little as a few months, as much as several years, or on average 3 years.

I know hindsight is perfect vision, but if I knew two years ago what I know now there is a very good chance that I would not be on cancer's death row awaiting execution. Unfortunately, on cancer's death row you may get a stay of execution (remission) but no pardon. It is a pity that nobody gave me this book to read two years ago (impossible I know).

Being very annoyed, I decided that I would find out more about the "enemy within" and why I was ignorant of the symptoms and risks. After a few months I found out that I was not alone in my ignorance as research had shown that around 50% of men in the "at risk" category are also ignorant of the symptoms and risks.

I also found out that a lot of men ignore "problems down below" as it could be seen as something wrong with their masculinity, a taboo subject men do not want to talk about. And, when men see the words "prostate cancer" they switch off as they perceive it to be exclusively an old man's disease, just like I did.

I also discovered that the UK Department of Health will not run a national screening programme for prostate cancer like it does for cervical and breast cancer in women. Because of this decision, the UK Department of Health does not provide any public information broadcasts on TV or Radio about the symptoms and risks of the disease.

Also, only a small number of GP surgeries offer a "well man clinic" service that screens men when they reach the "at risk" age (40 years for African Caribbean and 45 years for white European).

Based on these discoveries, it is clear to me that men need to become more aware as well as take control of their own screening programme, because contrary to belief, the NHS does not look after the nation's health.

As a consequence, your health is your responsibility whether you are a man or a woman.

After this journey of "enlightenment" I have decided to spend a major part of the time I have remaining leading a campaign with the goal of providing greater awareness of the symptoms and risks of prostate cancer.

I hope that reading this book will help towards meeting this goal. Remember ignorance is bliss but ignorance kills.

It is important to note that many of the symptoms mentioned in this book are not life threatening and if prostate cancer, like other cancers, is diagnosed early enough it is curable.

Another reassuring point is that more men die with prostate cancer than those that die from it.

This said, my simple message is don't ignore the symptoms and risks.

Yours sincerely

Doug Gray

Content

Foreword	1
Acknowledgements	5
1. Introduction	7
2. Symptoms & Risks	11
3. Dinky & Donky	15
4. The Prostate Specific Antigen (PSA) Test	17
5. The Digital Rectum Examination (DRE)	19
6. The Risk Management Programme	21
7. Minimising the Risks	25
8. Taking Control	29
9. The Greater Awareness Campaign	37
10. What to Do Next	41
11. The Male Reproductive System	43
12. Prostate Cancer Treatments	49

13. Author's Personal Opinion	53
14. Facts and Supporting Information	67
15. Support Organisations	71
Epilogue	73
About the Author	75
Glossary	77
Information Sources	79

Foreword

The inspiration for the title and cover photograph of this book came from the Author's privilege to listen to a talk by Consultant Urologist Surgeon, David Baxter-Smith, on prostate cancer. During the talk he raised is right hand with his index finger extended and said, quote: "It has been estimated that during my career this finger had been up the backsides of 40,000 men, 4 of which were in the House of Lords".

An attractive woman posing as a doctor on the front cover has been chosen to help alleviate the concern some men have regarding a Digital Rectum Examination (medical term for a gloved and lubricated doctor's finger probing up the backside) being an unpleasant experience (it probably is for a doctor).

Although prostate cancer is a male disease, it is important that women also read this book as they can often persuade their partner, father, brothers, uncles, male colleagues and friends to take action, thus preventing them being one of the 10,000 unnecessary deaths each year.

Once read, **this book should not to be left on a shelf gathering dust**. Instead, it should be **gifted or loaned to another person**, male or female, to increase awareness and potentially save men's lives.

To measure the book's effectiveness, as well as recording its journey in meeting the book's objective, the following table is provided to enter the date the book is read and add any appropriate remarks before gifting the book to another person.

Reader	Date Read	Remarks
1		
2		
3		
4		
5		
6		
7		
8		
9		
10		
11		
12		
13		
14		
15		
16		
17		
18		
19		
20		

Acknowledgements

There are too many individuals and organisations for the Author to acknowledge their contributions in making this book possible. Nevertheless, he would like to acknowledge and thank the following individuals and organisations:

Individuals

David Baxter-Smith:	Consultant Urological Surgeon and President of the Kidderminster Cancer Support Group www.kidderminsterpcsg.com
Sandy Tyndale-Biscoe:	Chairman of the Prostate Cancer Support Federation www.prostatecancerfederation.org.uk
Peter Hosking:	Chairman of the Torbay Prostate Support Association (PSA)
Graham Fulford:	Graham Fulford Charity www.guidestar.org.uk
Aleksandra:	A family member who posed for the front cover photograph
Christopher Halls:	Cover Artwork & Design
	Minds Eye Design: www.mindseyedesign.co.uk

Organisations

The UK Department of Health
The UK National Screening Committee
Cancer Research www.cancerresearchuk.org
The Prostate Cancer Charity www.prostate-cancer.org.uk

Chapter 1

Introduction

This introductory chapter has been produced to serve as an overview of the content of each chapter in this book.

For those men and women who easily get bored when reading, the most important information and essential reading is contained in the Letter from the Author, the Foreword and Chapters 2 through 8.

Chapters 9 through 15 contain useful background information for increased knowledge about prostate cancer and how the reader can help spread the "greater awareness of the symptoms and risks of prostate cancer" message.

Chapter 2: Symptoms & Risks

An overview of the early warning symptoms and the risks of developing prostate cancer.

Chapter 3: Dinky & Donky

A wee rhyming tale extolling the virtue of recognising the symptoms and risks.

Chapter 4: The Prostate Specific Antigen (PSA) Test

The reason why a PSA blood test is required as part of helping to diagnose the possibility of prostate cancer.

Chapter 5: The Digital Rectum Examination (DRE)

An explanation of why a DRE is required as part of helping to diagnose the possibility of the disease.

Chapter 1: Introduction

Chapter 6: The Risk Management Programme

An explanation of the Prostate Cancer Risk Management Programme (PCRMP) intended to be followed by GPs when men request a PSA test, so that they can make an "informed decision" before proceeding with the test.

Chapter 7: Minimising the Risks

What men can do to help minimise the risks of developing prostate cancer.

Chapter 8: Taking Control

A method of combining the Risks, DRE and PSA tests into a personal screening programme.

Chapter 9: The Greater Awareness Campaign

The author explains details of the greater awareness campaign that commenced in July 2009 and will hopefully continue until the Department of Health decides to implement national screening for prostate cancer.

Chapter 10: What to Do Next

Provided here are details of the opportunities available to increase the effectiveness of the greater awareness campaign thus helping to save men's lives and extend the life expectancy of men who develop prostate cancer.

Chapter 11: The Male Reproductive System

A practical and easily understood description of the male reproductive system.

Chapter 12: Prostate Cancer Treatments

Descriptions of the procedures available to treat localised, locally advanced and advance prostate cancer.

Chapter 13: Author's Personal Opinion

Here, the Author provides the reasons why he strongly believes the UK Department of Health is highly unlikely to implement national screening for prostate cancer and is also highly unlikely to provide greater public awareness using media public information broadcasts and other appropriate means.

Chapter 14: Facts and Supporting Information

Important information covering the key facts relating to the disease and some useful supporting information indicating why the Department of Health is highly unlikely to introduce national screening for prostate cancer.

Chapter 15: Support Organisations

A list of organisations dedicated to the support of men with prostate cancer and their families.

Chapter 2

Symptoms & Risks

Symptoms

Contrary to belief, prostate cancer is not just an "old man's" disease as approximately 20% of men diagnosed with the disease are aged 65 years or younger. For example, the author knows one angry man who was diagnosed at the age of 41 and several diagnosed in their early 50s.

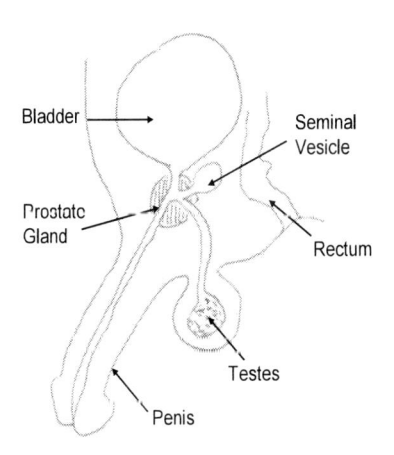

Figure 1: Prostate Gland and Surrounding Organs

Figure 1 above shows the prostate gland and surrounding organs. A normal healthy prostate gland in a young man is about the size of a walnut.

Chapter 2: Symptoms & Risks

However, at around the age of 50 the prostate gland can start to enlarge and progressively get larger as a man's age increases.

This enlargement can restrict the flow of urine from the bladder and thus cause one or more of the following changes in passing urine:

- **Reduced flow:** It takes longer to empty the bladder.
- **Hesitancy:** Waiting a while before urine flows.
- **Leaking**: A small leak after finishing.
- **Increased Frequency:** Visits to the toilet in the night.
- **Urgency:** A need to get to the toilet quickly.
- **Poor Emptying:** A feeling of not quite emptying the bladder.

Most men who develop the above symptoms do not have prostate cancer but have a benign (non-cancerous) enlargement of the prostate. However, some of these growths are found to be cancerous.

Fortunately, some of these cancers are slow growing (known as "pussycats") and not life threatening. For example, it is often quoted that more men die with prostate cancer than those that die from it.

This said, a number of these cancers are very aggressive (know as "tigers") and life threatening. For this reason it is important that men do not ignore the symptoms and risks.

Important: Unfortunately, the most important symptom is no symptoms at all, hence the reason why men are urged to take control of their own screening in the absence of a national screening programme (see chapter 8).

Chapter 2: Symptoms & Risks

Because the prostate is a male sex gland some studies have indicated that changes in sexual function could signal possible prostate problems, such as:

- Lack of libido/sex drive
- Erectile dysfunction (poor erection)
- Reduced ejaculate

If the cancer spreads to other parts of the body, other symptoms can develop.

The most common site for the cancer to spread is to one or more bones, especially the pelvis, lower spine and hips.

Affected bones can become painful and tender. Sometimes the first symptoms to develop are from secondary tumours in bones.

Risks

- Age
- Genes
- Diet
- Damage
- Tall
- Overweight
- Exposure

Age: African Caribbean men are at risk when aged 40 years or more and white European men when aged 45 years or more.

Chapter 2: Symptoms & Risks

Genes

Men are at risk if:

- Their father had/has prostate cancer
- Their brother had/has prostate cancer
- Their sister had a certain type of breast cancer
- They are African Caribbean

Unfortunately, the NHS does not operate any form of genetic screening for men at risk of prostate cancer.

As a consequence men will need to rely on being informed of the risk by family members who have developed the disease and tell those in their family (brothers and sons for prostate cancer and sisters for breast cancer) who will be at risk if they unfortunately develop the disease.

Diet: A diet high in animal fats and low in fruit and vegetables is believed to increase the risk.

Damage: Damage to the prostate gland through, for example, invasive procedures or objects inserted in the rectum.

Height: Some research has indicated that taller men (taller than 6 feet) have a higher risk.

Overweight: Men who are overweight or obese are at greater risk.

Exposure: Men exposed to the metal cadmium may also be at risk.

Chapter 3

Dinky & Donky

Dinky and Donky drank lots of tea,
to see who could wee furthest up a tree

When they were boys it wasn't very high,
but when they were men it nearly reached the sky

At middle age it went well up the tree,
but later Donky couldn't wee above his knee

Not only that he took ages to finish,
with dribbles and shakes until his wee diminished

Standing alone and weeing to one side,
Dinky was saddened that Donky had died

So don't be an ASS and don't be a DINKY,
tell your friends when their wee is WONKY

And if you have a problem with your wee,
get off your ass and see your GP

The morale of this "wee" rhyming tale is:
"Don't Ignore the Signs"

Chapter 4

The Prostate Specific Antigen (PSA) Test

The Prostate Specific Antigen (PSA) blood test is a very simple test that measures very accurately the levels of antigens (proteins) secreted from the prostate gland into the blood. As the antigens are produced solely by the prostate, raised levels can be a good indicator of cancer.

Unfortunately, even though the PSA blood test is very accurate, actual results vary from individual to individual based on a number of factors such as age, health, sexual activity, exercise, stress, medication, constipation, etc. Because of these variations, "false negatives" and "false positives" often occur as a result of interpretation.

However, cancer is unlikely if a PSA level is not raised and as a result no immediate action is needed, although sometimes further tests may be required to confirm the result.

If a PSA level is slightly raised it may not be cancer, but more tests might be needed, including more PSA tests. If the PSA level is very high (the Author's PSA level when admitted into hospital was 111) this is a very clear indication of prostate cancer requiring urgent treatment.

Also, there are two types of prostate cancer, "pussycats" that grow very slowly and can be no threat to life and "tigers" that are very aggressive and life threatening.

Because of the possibility of "false negatives" and "false positives" the NHS has put in place a Risk Management Programme (see chapter 6) that all GPs must follow.

Chapter 4: The Prostate Specific Antigen (PSA) Test

This programme is aimed to advise a man who requests a PSA test what he must consider and decide before taking, or not taking, the test.

The benefits of PSA testing are:
- It may be reassuring if the test result is normal.
- It may give an indication of cancer before symptoms develop.
- It may find cancer at an early stage when treatments could be of benefit.
- If treatment is successful, the worst possible outcomes of more advanced cancer, including death, are avoided.
- Even if the cancer is more advanced and treatment is less successful, it will usually extend life.

The limitations of PSA testing are:
- It can miss cancer and provide false reassurance.
- It may lead to unnecessary worry and medical tests when there is no cancer.
- It cannot tell the difference between slow-growing (pussycat) and fast-growing (tiger) cancers.
- It may make you worry by finding slow-growing cancers that may never cause any symptoms or shorten your life.

Chapter 5

The Digital Rectum Examination (DRE)

The title of this book "A finger up your...." adequately describes a Digital Rectum Examination (DRE). Contrary to what some men may believe a DRE is not a painful experience.

If men have not had the pleasure of experiencing a DRE the procedure is very simple. Men are asked by the doctor to lie on their side on an examination bed facing away from the doctor, slide their trousers and underpants down their legs and bring their knees up to their chest exposing their buttocks and rectum.

The doctor puts on a latex glove, lubricates the index finger and then inserts it into the rectum. The doctor then moves the finder around inside feeling the texture of the flesh surrounding the prostate gland which is located a short distance inside the anal passage.

If an enlargement, roughness or hard textured flesh is detected this could indicate a problem with the prostate. If the doctor suspects a problem the patient may be asked to take a Prostate Specific Antigen (PSA) blood test (see chapter 4) and have an ultrasound image scan of the prostate at their nearest hospital.

Unfortunately, even if the DRE reveals no abnormalities this does not necessarily mean men are free from prostate cancer. This is because a DRE examination is dependent to a large extent on the experience of the doctor to detect any abnormalities.

Chapter 5: The Digital Rectum Examination (DRE)

Also, a very small area of hard cancerous cells is very difficult to detect by a human finger. In addition, if DREs are performed by different clinicians at different times, comparing and referencing results accurately would be difficult.

Fortunately, technology is already here to allow the design, development and production of a low cost mechanical DRE that could electronically record the size and texture of the prostate in all dimensions along the length of the anal passage in which it is inserted.

As no human interpretation is involved, the electronic record would be more accurate and could be easily compared with subsequent mechanical DREs to identify "rate of change" abnormalities. Ideally, such an apparatus would be used by Doctors and qualified nurses in GP surgeries.

Unfortunately, even though mechanical DREs do exist they are very expensive and not widely available thus preventing widespread use by GPs where they are more importantly needed.

This said, a DRE is a useful examination, especially if a man is experiencing any of the passing of urine symptoms mentioned in chapter 2, but taken alone it is not conclusive and therefore further tests are required.

Chapter 6

The Risk Management Programme

As mentioned in chapter 4, the NHS has put in place a Prostate Cancer Risk Management Programme (PCRMP) that all GPs must follow. This programme has been provided to advise men requesting a PSA blood test what they must consider before deciding whether to take, or not take, the test.

The reason for this advice is because the results of a PSA blood test could indicate "false negatives" and "false positives". In other words, the test could be negative when prostate cancer is present or the test could be positive when prostate cancer is not present.

Therefore, the PCRMP lists all the benefits and risks associated with taking a PSA blood test thus allowing men to make in informed choice.

For example, if a PSA level is raised, a prostate biopsy may be needed to check for cancer. This means taking samples from the prostate via the rectum. Many men find this is an embarrassing and uncomfortable experience and some describe it as painful, although local anaesthetics help. Sometimes the biopsy may lead to complications (such as blood in the semen or urine) or infection.

About 2 out of 3 men who have a prostate biopsy will not have prostate cancer. However, biopsies can miss some cancers and the patient may not know for sure that he does not have cancer after a clear result.

Chapter 6: The Risk Management Programme

The main treatment procedures for dealing with prostate cancer are described in chapter 12. Like all procedures there are risks and possible complications, such as serious infection, incontinence and erectile dysfunction (impotence).

The likelihood of complications depends on the chosen treatment and most importantly, the expertise of the surgeon and the age of the treatment equipment used. Note: Because the latest generation of equipment is expensive it is rarely purchased by the NHS until usage is widespread and costs have come down.

Interesting, it is mainly because of the risk of complications mentioned above that the Department of Health will not implement a national screening programme for prostate cancer.

As a consequence, only those men who have been fortunate enough to have been made aware of the symptoms and risks of prostate cancer actually request the PSA test from their GP, hence the need for greater awareness.

Cautionary Tale:

One of the Author's brothers, when he was informed that he was at risk of developing prostate cancer, took a PSA blood test which showed a higher than normal level. Having been told he needed to have a biopsy, he asked his older brother (the author) whether it was painful.

The Author told him he only experienced slight pain each time a sample was taken and suffered no bleeding or urinary problems afterwards.

The Author's brother went ahead with the biopsy, which was painful but it confirmed he had prostate cancer.

Chapter 6: The Risk Management Programme

Fortunately, it was localised prostate cancer and curable, unlike his older brother's cancer.

The moral of this tale is "It is better to be safe than sorry".

Chapter 7

Minimising the Risks

Obviously, prevention is better than cure. Even though prevention is possible, it is an extreme measure that the vast majority of men would not be willing to take.

For example, cervical cancer in women is linked to sexual activity. Proof of this fact is that the incidence of cervical cancer in women of holy orders, such as Nuns, is practically non-existent

Prostate cancer in men is also linked to sexual activity. For example, men who have become Eunuchs are sexually inactive and as such the incidence of prostate cancer is again practically non-existent.

Therefore, the only way to prevent the disease is to become a Eunuch at puberty or have a varied and active sex life until the "at risk" age and then go hang gliding without a hang glider.

The risks of developing prostate cancer as already mentioned are listed below in order of importance.

- **Age**
- **Genes**
- **Diet**
- **Damage**
- **Tall**
- **Overweight**
- **Exposure**

Chapter 7: Minimising the Risks

Age: The biggest risk is age as the likelihood of developing prostate cancer starts at around 40 years of age for African Caribbean men and 45 years of age for white European men.

As there is nothing we can do about growing older (unless a man's life unfortunately ends before this age) he must start to recognise that he is at risk and take appropriate steps to check his health regularly. Chapter 8, "Taking Control" will explain in more detail the appropriate steps men can take.

Genes: As mentioned previously, the second highest risk after age is family genes. Because of the "taboo" associated with prostate cancer (the stigma of a disease that can seriously affect a man's libido and sexual function) men from older generations very rarely discuss their condition and tell anyone of its symptoms and risks, even family members.

Therefore, it is essential that men find out details of their family's health problems as this knowledge will indicate risks for a number of diseases, not only prostate cancer. Unfortunately, if a man is the oldest, it is unlikely he will get any genetic risk warning and therefore it will be up to him to ensure he checks his health more rigorously.

Diet: Without preaching too much, diet is extremely important. There is no doubt that people who have a healthy diet, as well as exercise regularly live longer, have greater immunity to a number of diseases and recover faster when they unfortunately get ill.

With regard to diet, a number of studies have already indicated that a diet high in dairy products such as milk, cheese, butter and red meat (beef) increase the risk of prostate cancer.

Chapter 7: Minimising the Risks

For example, men in Asia have a low incidence of prostate cancer compared with men in Northern Europe. Interestingly, Japanese men have the lowest incident of prostate cancer.

From various information sources there are regular claims that the following food stuffs help prevent and also slow down the growth of prostate cancer.

Tomatoes: In the form of Ketchup, puree, canned, mashed, cooked, etc., not raw tomatoes as the body is unable to extract the beneficial properties from the skin.

Asparagus:

Broccoli:

Soya Milk:

Pomegranate Juice:

Green Tea:

Therefore, it could be beneficial to introduce these food stuffs regularly as part of a "five a day" diet. Interestingly, green tea is drunk a lot in Asia. Also, because of the amount of fish Japanese men eat it seems common sense and logical to eat more oily fish.

Supplements of selenium and vitamin D (if you cannot get 15 minutes of sunshine a day) are considered beneficial.

Further information and advice on a preventative diet can be found in the book titled "Prostate Cancer" by Professor Jane Plant, a book that looks at a number of worldwide studies and research that strongly indicates a diet rich in dairy products causes both breast cancer and prostate cancer.

With regard to exercise, the more physically fit the body is, combined with a good diet, the better it is at repairing damage.

For example, cancer can develop when damaged cells are replaced by new cells which are not perfect replicas.

In summary, it is common sense and logic that a good diet, combined with a balanced exercise regime to increase strength and stamina will help increase longevity and provide greater immunity to all diseases in general.

Damage: Men should refrain from any activity that may cause damage to the prostate gland. As already mentioned, a sensible diet and exercise regime should improve the body's ability to replace any damaged cells with healthy cells if and when damage occurs.

Tall: Like age there is nothing that can be done to minimise the risk other than to be aware of the risk.

Overweight: A sensible diet and exercise regime will obviously help keep weight under control.

Exposure: Cadmium inhalation can be an occupational hazard associated with industrial processes such as metal plating and the production of nickel-cadmium batteries, pigments, plastics, and other synthetics.

Environmental exposure is primarily the result of burning fossil fuels and municipal waste and subsequent exposure to cadmium in contaminated food and water.

Tobacco smoking is the most significant source of cadmium exposure. On average, smokers have 4 to 5 times higher blood cadmium concentrations than non-smokers.

It is therefore common sense for men to take adequate precautions when working in hazardous industries, be aware of the risks (if any) in their local environment and if they smoke, stop smoking.

Chapter 8

Taking Control

From reading chapters 4, 5, 6 and this chapter, men will have the necessary information and knowledge to take control of their own screening programme until the Department of Health decides (if they ever do) to implement a national screening programme for prostate cancer.

Men already in the "At Risk" age group of 40 years or more if African Caribbean or aged 45 years or more if white European can check if they are at additional risk by simply ticking the risk factors as they apply to them in the table below.

Important: Please produce a copy of the risk factor table below on a piece of paper and don't mark this page as the book will need to be passed on to keep delivering the greater awareness message.

Risk Factors	Tick
Father has/had prostate cancer	
Brother/Brothers has/had prostate cancer	
Sister has/had breast cancer	
Diet high in animal fats and diary products	
Diet low in fruit and vegetables	
Very tall (higher than 6 feet)	
Overweight	

The more risk factors ticked the greater the risk and the higher up the list the ticks are, the greater the risk.

Chapter 8: Taking Control

Note: Symptoms have not been included as these are obvious signs of a possible problem that must be checked out.

Because the most important symptom of prostate cancer can be "no symptoms at all" it is advisable that men start their own screening programme when they reach the "At Risk" age group, especially if they have ticked any of the risk factors listed previously.

The basic benchmark for the personal screening programme is the DRE and the PSA blood test.

The first step is for men to make an appointment with their GP.

At the appointment men must explain that they have decided to carry out their own prostate cancer screening programme because there is no national screening programme or a GP "well man clinic" (if applicable) that includes testing for prostate cancer. For these reasons a DRE and a PSA blood test is requested.

Unfortunately, some GPs can misinterpret the Prostate Cancer Risk Management Programme (see chapter 6) and have wrongly refused to take a PSA blood test when requested.

Therefore, it is important that men remain firm with their GP if he or she tries to dissuade them from taking the test, or refuses to do the test.

If he or she refuses, men must remind them that it is their right to have the test and if they still refuse, they will write an official complaint as well as change their doctor.

Assuming the GP agrees to the PSA blood test, a follow up appointment with the surgery nurse for a blood sample will usually be required.

The next stage is for the GP to carry out a DRE.

Chapter 8: Taking Control

As a DRE will stimulate the prostate gland men should refrain from any activity that may stimulate the prostate gland, such as exercising heavily and/or ejaculating though sexual activity in the period 48 hours before providing the PSA blood sample.

Also, when the DRE is carried out request the GP to provide a rating of the size, roughness and hardness of the flesh around the prostate using the following rating scores:

- Size (1 small, 5 large)
- Roughness (1 smooth, 5 rough)
- Hardness (1 soft, 5 hard)

Explain that this rating will be used as a benchmark for subsequent DREs if required.

Because the interpretation of a DRE can vary between clinicians it is advisable that men ask the same GP to do this test, if and when it needs to be repeated.

Normally, the results of a PSA test will be available within 3 working days after the blood sample is taken. If men have not been notified of the result within this period, they should contact their surgery for the result. It is important that they obtain the actual result and not accept being told it is in within normal ranges.

Once men have obtained their DRE ratings and their PSA blood test result they now have a screening benchmark for future reference.

Assuming these results are normal, the next stage is to repeat the DRE and PSA tests 6 months later. The reason these need to be repeated is that the **"Rate of Change"** is the most significant indicator that all is well or that something could be seriously wrong.

Chapter 8: Taking Control

Graph 1 below shows the maximum acceptable PSA levels versus men's ages extrapolated from a laboratory blood test report which indicates age 40-49, PSA <2.5, 50-59 PSA <3.5, 60-69 PSA <4.5 and 70-79 PSA <6.5.

For example, if a man's aged is 49 and his PSA level is 1.5 (lower than the upper limit of 2.5) he is within an acceptable range. However, if his level 6 months later rises to 2.4 he is still within an acceptable range but he could be at risk.

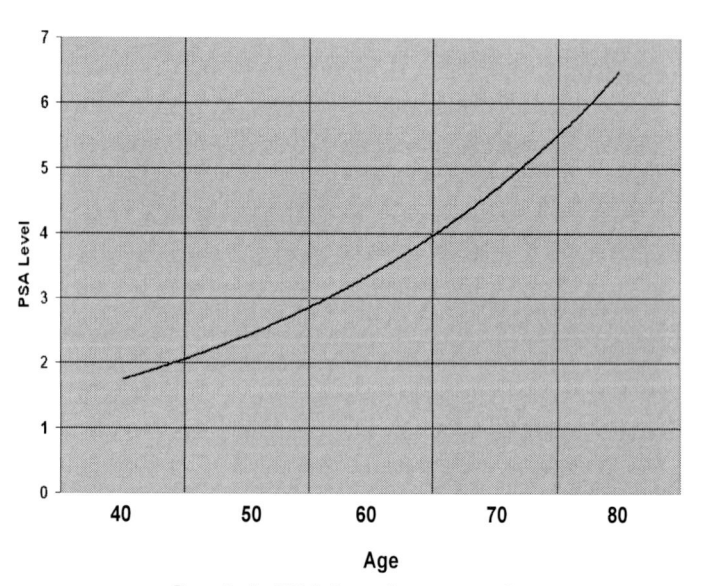

Graph 1: PSA Levels versus Age

If this was the case it would be advisable for him to take another PSA blood test 3 months later and look at the trend. If it has not risen or gone down everything should be OK. However, if the trend is still upwards his GP needs to be consulted.

Chapter 8: Taking Control

Similarly, if his DRE ratings were 1 for size, 1 for roughness and 1 for hardness this is a good indicator that all is well.

As there are no accurate measures for size, roughness and hardness, the ratings from this examination are solely based on the GP's finger sensitivity, expertise and interpretation.

Also, as there are no measures against age, other than the prostate gland normally gets larger as men get older the ratings again are solely based on the GP's finger sensitivity, expertise and interpretation.

This said, a GP should be able to determine if a prostate is abnormally enlarged and if the flesh around the prostate is rough and hard, which indicates a possible problem that needs further investigation.

However, with regard to the previous DRE example, if the ratings carried out by the same GP 6 months later show ratings of 2, 2 and 2 respectively, this also indicates that something could be wrong. Again, it would be advisable to carry out another DRE 3 months later.

Conversely, if the second DRE and PSA tests show no change this is a positive indicator that all is well and that all is needed is to repeat the tests every 12 months.

From the above example it can be seen that the "rate of change" results from both the DRE and PSA test, when combined, are a powerful indicator that all is well or that something could be wrong.

Research in the USA has shown that the rate at which a PSA level doubles is also a good indicator of whether a prostate cancer is a "pussycat" or a "tiger". For example, the shorter the doubling time the more aggressive the cancer and the longer the doubling time the less aggressive the cancer.

33

Chapter 8: Taking Control

In addition to the DRE and PSA test, it may be beneficial for men to observe and take note from time to time their sexual performance in terms of their libido, erectile strength and amount of ejaculate.

Any changes could indicate a problem, especially reduced ejaculate because approximately 25% is produced by the prostate and 75% by the seminal vesicle (see chapter 11) which is very close to the prostate gland.

Important: Please do not write on the table and steps page in this book as it needs to be gifted to other people to increase awareness of the symptoms and risks of prostate cancer.

Therefore, it is recommended that all men who decide to implement their own screening programme reproduce the following table on a separate piece of paper for the purpose of recording and comparing results.

Chapter 8: Taking Control

Test Date	Elapsed Time Since Previous Test (Weeks)	DRE Prostate Size Rating	DRE Prostate Roughness Rating	DRE Prostate Hardness Rating	PSA Level

Step 1: Arrange GP Appointment

Step 2: Request a DRE with its ratings followed by a PSA blood test. If within acceptable ranges move to step 3. If not, consult GP for further tests

Step 3: Record results on table (replica of above)

Step 4: Repeat DRE and PSA tests 6 months later and record results on table

Step 5: Compare results against previous results. If no change, or lowering of readings, repeat tests 12 months later. If within ranges but levels have increased repeat tests again 3 months later. If results continue to rise and/or exceed limits consult GP

Chapter 9

The Greater Awareness Campaign

Figure 2 below summarises the problem and indicates why a greater public awareness campaign of the symptoms and risks of prostate cancer is needed.

Sources
Government
Media
Family & Friends

Public Awareness

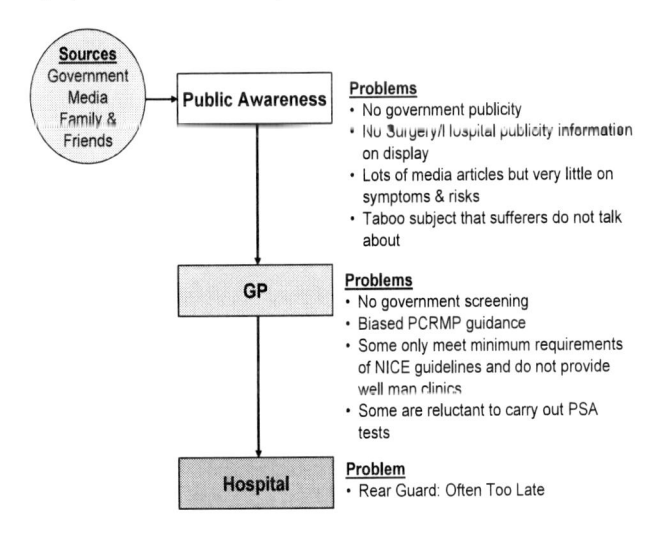

Problems
- No government publicity
- No Surgery/Hospital publicity information on display
- Lots of media articles but very little on symptoms & risks
- Taboo subject that sufferers do not talk about

GP

Problems
- No government screening
- Biased PCRMP guidance
- Some only meet minimum requirements of NICE guidelines and do not provide well man clinics
- Some are reluctant to carry out PSA tests

Hospital

Problem
- Rear Guard: Often Too Late

Figure 2: Reasons for Lack of Public Awareness

For example, the author of this book believes that if he knew two years ago what he knows now, there is a very good chance that he would not have advanced prostate cancer.

Chapter 9: The Greater Awareness Campaign

Even though he classed himself as being reasonably intelligent and well informed on most matters, the reason why he did not know two years ago what he knows now is that he did not find any information readily available to the public on prostate cancer that may have triggered him to request tests at his local GP surgery. Interestingly, media stories on prostate cancer (Newspapers, Radio, TV) very rarely tell you what symptoms to look out for.

In addition, if you go to your local GP surgery you will probably not see any prostate cancer information posters on the notice board or leaflets that you could take away (definitely the case in the Author's surgery).

Also, because of the 'taboo' associated with prostate problems, sufferers very rarely talk about their experiences with family, friends and colleagues, which again does not help increase awareness.

Another problem is that the words "Prostate Cancer" on leaflets is often instinctively ignored my men because it is perceived as solely an old man's disease. This perception is not helped as these leaflets (if lucky enough to find one) often shows an old man with a grey beard as the sufferer, when it is the men aged between 40 and 60 that are more likely to be unaware of the symptoms and risks.

These are probably the main reasons why very few men actually know what symptoms to look out for and know what factors increase the risk of developing prostate cancer, even though most of us know someone who has, or has had, the disease.

However, the overriding reason why men are less aware of prostate cancer, as mentioned several times previously, is because the Department of Health will not implement a national screening programme or provide greater public awareness of the symptoms and risks of the disease.

Chapter 9: The Greater Awareness Campaign

Recognising this lack of knowledge, there is definitely an urgent need to increase awareness of the symptoms and risks of prostate cancer in order to save lives and increase life expectancy.

As a consequence of trying to meet this urgent need, the Author of this book has tasked himself with the following objectives as a steering group member of the Derriford Prostate Support Group to:

1. Increase greater public awareness of the symptoms and risks of prostate cancer
2. Promote the need for men to take ownership of their own prostate cancer screening programme
3. Promote the introduction and benefits of national population screening for prostate cancer
4. Carry out prostate cancer patient research in areas that will assist with objectives 1, 2 & 3.
5. Identify areas that will help early diagnosis of prostate cancer, differentiate between the "tiger" and "pussycat" cancers and promote them as areas of research to other appropriate organisations
6. Work with/support and/or join as appropriate other organisations with similar objectives

The reason why this book has been written is to help meet objectives 1, 2 and 3.

Chapter 10

What To Do Next

There are a number of ways the reader of this book can contribute to the greater awareness of prostate cancer campaign. Some examples are as follows:

1. Read this book and then gift it to another person so that they can do the same (Thank You)

2. Inform all family, friends, colleagues, acquaintances, as appropriate (male and female) and tell them about the book and the web sites that have addition information such as the loveyourprostate,co.uk web site and those listed in the Acknowledgements.

3. If the reader has been motivated by this book to get more involved, then consider:

    a. Joining a local Prostate Cancer Support Group and become an active member of the committee (you do not need to be suffering from prostate cancer, be old or be a man)

    b. Raising money for one of the Charities or Prostate Cancer Support Groups

4. If a member of an organisation, club, society, etc., suggest that the committee invites a speaker from the local Prostate Cancer Support Group to talk about the disease.

5. **MOST IMPORTANT:** If a man is in the "at risk" age group they must take control of their own screening programme.

Chapter 11

The Male Reproductive System

To simplify the description of the male reproductive system a block diagram using easily understood mechanical and electrical devices has been used. This can be seen in Figure 3 on the next page.

Basically, the system comprises a number of fluid stores, fluid pumps, ducts and a senor probe. Not shown is the processor (brain) that controls the operation of the system.

The main component parts of the reproductive system are the prostate gland (A), the seminal vesicle (B) the bulbourethral glands (C) and the testes (D).

Although not an essential part of the reproductive system, the bladder is depicted as liquid storage tank (1) and the penis is depicted as sensor probe (10).

- The prostrate gland (A) comprises a valve (2), an Alkaline Fluid Store (3) and a Pump (5)
- The seminal vesicle (B) comprises a nutrient fluid store (4)
- The bulbourethral glands (C) comprise a lubricating fluid store (8) and a pump (6)
- The testes (D) comprise a fertiliser store (9) and a pump (7)

The dark lines are fluid ducts and the arrows show the direction of fluid flow.

When the reproductive system is not in operation all pumps are inoperative and valve (2) is open.

43

Chapter 11: The Male Reproductive System

Also, all fluid stores are full, assuming sufficient time for replenishment since the system was last used.

From sexual arousal to ejaculation of semen the following events take place.

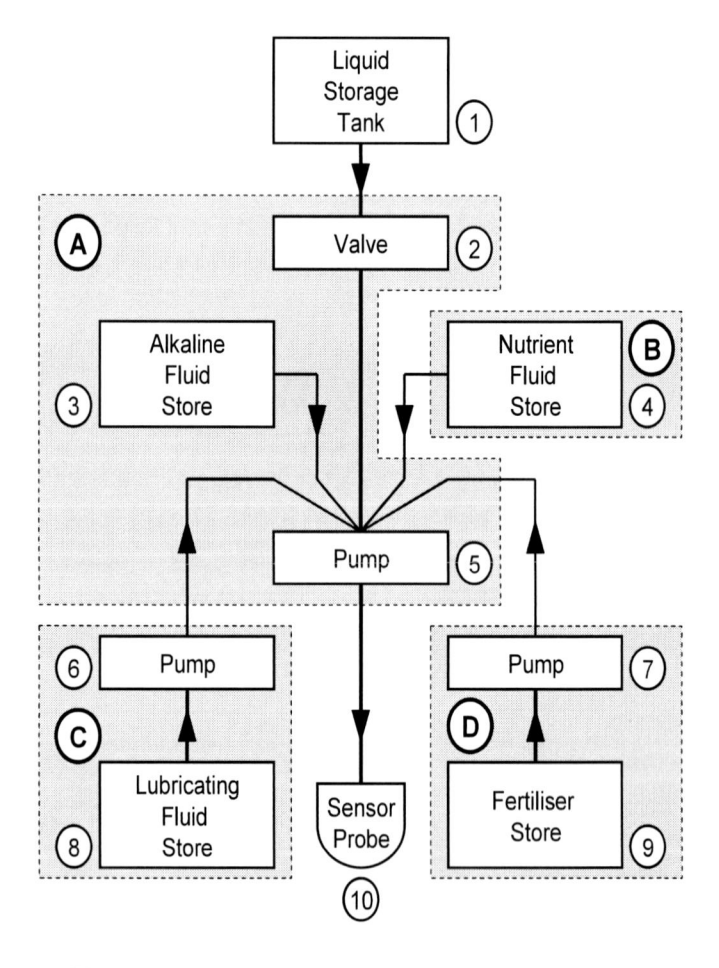

Figure 3: Male Reproductive System Block Diagram

Chapter 11: The Male Reproductive System

Event 1: The penis (10) becomes erect and the surface area becomes more sensitive to stimulus.

Event 2: After sexual arousal reaches a high state, valve (2) is closed to prevent flow of urine from the bladder (1) and any semen flow into the bladder.

Also, the lubricating fluid (8) is secreted by pump (6) through the open pump (5) down the fluid duct to seep from the end of the penis (10).

Event 3: At the point of ejaculation, pump (7) become operational along with the main ejaculatory pump (5), to combine and force the nutrient (4) and alkaline fluids (3) along with sperm from the fertiliser store (9) out of the penis (10).

Event 4: After ejaculation has occurred, the penis becomes placid and the system returns back to its rest state to allow replenishment of the fluid stores to take place.

The ejaculated fluid discharged from the penis is known as semen and is a combination of the alkaline, nutrient and lubricating fluids as well as the sperm.

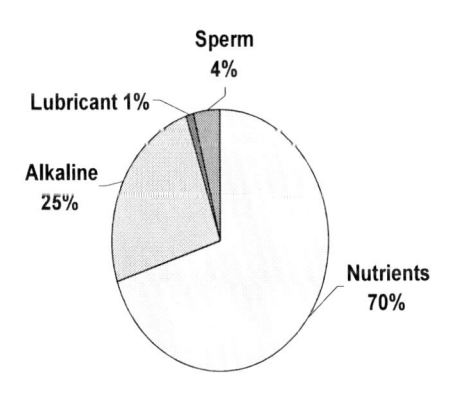

Chart 1: Constituent Parts of Semen

Chapter 11: The Male Reproductive System

The constituent parts of semen are shown in chart 1 on the previous page.

Although simplified, the constituent parts of semen basically comprise nutrients to feed the sperm on its journey (70%), an alkaline (antacid) solution (25%) to protect the sperm from the acidity of the virginal tract and a lubricant (1%) to cleanse and smooth the way for the semen along the urethra.

The actual sperm content represents less than 4% of the fluid ejaculated from the penis.

The prostate gland

The main function of the prostate is to store and secrete the alkaline fluid. The prostate also contains some smooth muscles that help expel semen during ejaculation.

A small amount of the alkaline fluid (less than 1%) includes proteolytic enzymes, prostatic acid phosaphatases and Prostate Specific Antigen (PSA). This fluid also contains zinc.

To work properly, the prostate needs male hormones (androgens), which are responsible for male sex characteristics. The most significant male hormone is testosterone, which is produced mainly by the testes. Some male hormones are produced in small amounts by the adrenal glands.

A healthy prostate is slightly larger than a walnut. It surrounds the urethra just below the urinary bladder and can be felt during a Digital Rectum Examination (DRE).

Table 1, on the following page describes the four zones and the constitution of the zones as a percentage of the prostate as a whole.

Chapter 11: The Male Reproductive System

Zone	Constitution (%)	Description
Peripheral Zone (PZ)	Composes up to 70% of the normal prostate gland in young men	The sub-capsular portion of the posterior aspect of the prostate gland which surrounds the distal urethra. It is from this portion of the gland that more than 64% of prostatic cancers originate.
Central Zone (CZ)	Constitutes approximately 25% of the normal prostate gland	This zone surrounds the ejaculatory ducts. The central zone accounts for roughly 2.5% of prostate cancers although these cancers tend to be more aggressive and more likely to invade the seminal vesicles.
Transition Zone (TZ)	Responsible for 5% of the prostate volume at puberty.	Prostate cancer originates in this zone in roughly 34% of patients. The transition zone surrounds the proximal urethra and is the region of the prostate gland which grows throughout life and is responsible for the disease of benign prostatic enlargement.
Anterior fibro-muscular zone (or stroma)	Accounts for approximately 5% of the prostatic weight	This zone is usually devoid of glandular components, and composed only, as its name suggests, of muscle and fibrous tissue.

Table 1: Prostate Zones

The prostate gland has four distinct glandular regions, two of which arise from different segments of the prostatic urethra.

The Central Zone accounts for the most aggressive prostate cancers which are more likely to invade the seminal vesicles. Although this zone only represents approximately 2.5% of cancers compared with the Peripheral Zone which represents 64% of cancers, the actual percentage of the aggressive cancers compared with all life threatening cancers is higher because 34% of all growths (those mainly originating in the Transition Zone) are benign.

The seminal vesicles

The seminal vesicles are posterior to the urinary bladder and just above the prostate gland. About 65-75% of the semen originates from the seminal vesicles, which contain proteins, enzymes, fructose, mucus, vitamin C, flavins, phosphorylcholine and prostaglandins.

High fructose concentrations provide nutrient energy for the spermatozoa as they travel through the female reproductive system.

Chapter 12

Prostate Cancer Treatments

The earlier prostate cancer is diagnosed the greater the number of treatment options and the greater the success of a cure. Figure 4 below shows the treatment options available for the different stages of prostate cancer.

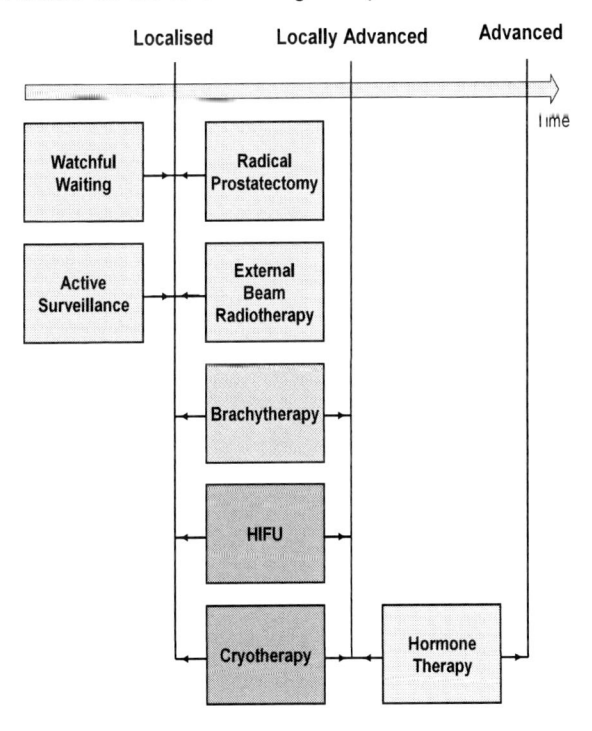

Figure 4: Treatment Options for Prostate Cancer Stages

Chapter 12: Prostate Cancer Treatments

However, lack of national screening and subsequent lack of awareness of the symptoms and hereditary gene risks, are causing prostate cancer to be diagnosed later than should normally occur.

As can be seen from figure 4 previously, there are seven treatment options available when the prostate cancer is at its earliest stage, with only three available when the cancer is locally advanced, Unfortunately, there is only one treatment available (hormone therapy) when the prostate cancer is advanced and incurable.

From the 2007/8 department of health statistics, Radical Prostatectomy is the most common treatment representing at 76% of all treatments (excluding Watchful Waiting, Active Surveillance and Hormone Therapy) for prostate cancer as can be seen from the pie chart in Chart 2 below.

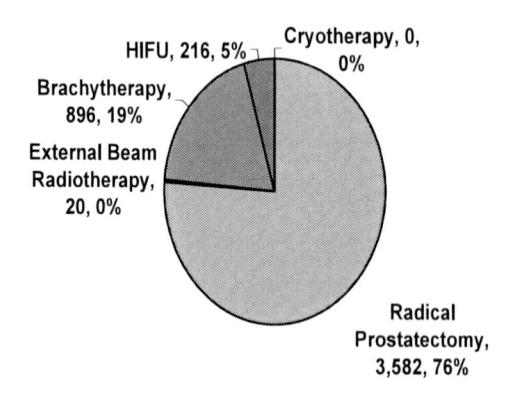

Chart 2: Treatments for Prostate Cancer 2007-8

Chapter 12: Prostate Cancer Treatments

As can been seen from the chart, Brachytheraphy is becoming a popular treatment for localised prostate cancer after its recent adoption by the NHS as is High Intensity Focussed Ultrasound (HIFU). Currently, Cryotheraphy is not available on the NHS.

Like all surgery there are associated risks. In the case of prostate cancer the greatest risks caused by surgery are complications such as serious infections, incontinence and lack of libido/erectile dysfunction.

For example, it is reported that after surgery up to 20% of Radical Prostatectomy procedures result in complications, which reduce to around 2% after further treatment of the complications.

It is expected that complications will reduce in the near future as robotic instruments operated by surgeons to minimise human error are used to carry out surgical procedures.

The risk of complications for both Low Dose Rate (LDR) and High Dose Rate (HDR) Brachytheraphy is <2% for incontinence and between 20-30% for impotence for men aged under 60 years. However, men with impotence respond well to Viagra.

Unfortunately, there is no significant historical data for the recent HIFU and Cryotherapy treatments to indicate the risk of complications.

Although not previously mentioned, there is a promising new treatment known as Photo Dynamic Therapy (PDT) in the USA which has been primarily used to treat skin cancer. However, PDT is being considered for deeper cancers such as prostate cancer. The way in which this therapy works is that a photo sensitive drug is introduced in such a way that it is absorbed by the cancer.

Chapter 12: Prostate Cancer Treatments

When the cancer cells are subsequently irradiated by infra-red light the cells are destroyed. The procedure uses probes inserted through the perineum in much the same way as Brachytherapy. However, the procedure as yet has not been approved by the Food and Drug Administration (FDA) of the USA for the treatment of prostate cancer.

In summary, the most important aspect of treatment is that the earlier the prostate cancer is diagnosed the greater the number of treatment options and the greater the success of a cure, thus saving lives and extending life expectancy.

Chapter 13

Author's Personal Opinion

7th September 2009

Dear Reader,

This is where I (the Author) get on my "Soap Box" and "Rant and Rave". However, before you start reading this chapter, please note that because it is a personal opinion from a very, very angry man, it is likely to offend some readers.

Why am I very, very angry? The answer is simple. I have incurable advanced prostate cancer, which will kill me sooner than later for no fault of my own. Yes, I could die in a hang gliding accident or get run over by a bus, but this is highly unlikely.

So whose fault is it? Some of you might think it is my fault for not being aware and taking control of my own health. However, my answer to this question is the Government on two counts and inconsistencies between GP practices.

Why? Because the Government, or should I say the Department of Health, have not introduced national screening for prostate cancer. If they had, my cancer would have been diagnosed early enough for me to have had treatment to cure the disease.

Chapter 13: Author's Personal Opinion

Also, if the Department of Health, with their "all singing and dancing" mega computer (both size and cost), had introduced a simple genetic screening programme for family members at risk, the type of breast cancer my sister developed two years ago would have resulted in me being automatically notified of my high risk of developing prostate cancer.

If (such significance for such a small word) my GP practice had run a "well man clinic" that recommended men over a certain age to take a PSA blood test, my prostate cancer would have been detected early enough for curative treatment.

Even though there is no national screening programme, no genetic screening programme or no "well man clinic" at my surgery, why did I not know about the symptoms and risks of prostate cancer?

Again the answer is simple. Because the Department of Health do not run a public awareness campaign (such a campaign would in effect result in national screening) to make men aware of the symptoms and risks of prostate cancer, I was unaware.

Surprisingly, I am not alone as recent research has shown that around 50% of "men at risk" are also unaware. The same research also indicated that the main sources of awareness for the other 50% were from family and friends and the media. Interestingly, GP surgeries, hospitals and health professionals ranked very low as awareness sources.

Chapter 13: Author's Personal Opinion

As a consequence, I am also annoyed that I can no longer:

- realise my dreams of seeing our grandchildren blossom into young adults
- continue to enjoy meeting people and making new friends
- eat out with my wife Janice and friends in the best of restaurants
- enjoy holidays with plenty of sun, sea, sand and socialising

I am also annoyed that my plans to rekindle my artistic talent and put all the pictures in my mind into oil on canvas have now become shattered dreams. I can go on and on with many more examples of what I'll miss because of my early departure.

Am I fearful of dying? No I'm not. What I am fearful of is the lingering death, doped up to the hilt with morphine with glimpses of loved ones, with tearful eyes, by my bedside when I briefly regain consciousness from my drug induced coma.

Maybe it would be better to go hang gliding without a hang glider or get run over by a bus.

Is the Department of Health ever going to introduce national screening for prostate cancer?

In my opinion the answer is definitely no. If any of you feel they will you are smoking opium.

Chapter 13: Author's Personal Opinion

Why? Again, the answer is very simple.

For example, my opinion is based on the following.

1. Older men have already made their financial contribution to the state and extending their life expectancy will cost the government a significant amount of money. In other words, this opportunity to save lives has a very poor return on investment.
2. Older men worth saving are the privileged few who already have private heath screening programmes as part of their employment or retirement package.

In addition, because of family history, vocations (such as health professionals) and those fortunate enough to have a GP who feels it necessary to screen men when they reach the "at risk" age, some men are more aware than others. Interestingly, the men at most risk, owing to lack of awareness, are blue collar workers.

Although many people believe that prostate cancer is an old man's disease, I know several men who were diagnosed in their early 50s and one very angry young man diagnosed at the age of 41.

Even though my belief that old men's lives are not worth saving (as far as the Government is concerned) may be considered extreme to some, the following logic explains this belief in more detail.

Chapter 13: Author's Personal Opinion

From the 2007 prostate cancer deaths graph below, approximately 7% of men die of prostate cancer before the retirement age of 65, which means 93% die aged 65 or over. Interestingly, 63% of the men that die are aged more than the average life expectancy of men, which is 77 years in the UK.

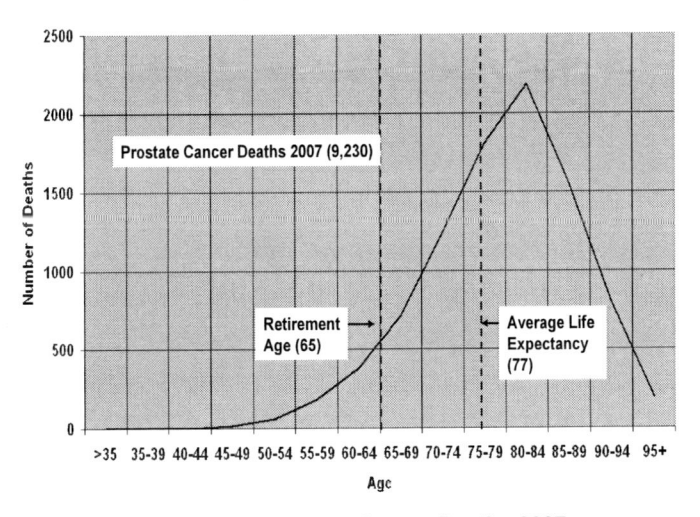

Graph 2: Prostate Cancer Deaths 2007

From a crude calculation based on the average old age pension of £7,800 pa, the annual cost for prescriptions and medical care (£1,500) and incidentals such as winter fuel payment, free bus travel, etc. (£700), the cost to the government of saving 2,000 lives each year (the reported number of lives that could be saved according to the recent European randomised study), is £20 million.

Chapter 13: Author's Personal Opinion

The cost of increasing the life expectancy of men by diagnosing prostate cancer earlier, using the same cost estimates as before and assuming that 35,000 men are diagnosed each year with prostate cancer of which another 8,000 die is approximately (35,000 - 8,000 x £10,000) = £270.0 Million per annum. This means national screening would cost the government nearly £300 million each year.

Most importantly, this expense does not include the additional NHS cost of setting up and running the national screening service, which would be significant.

Based on this financial model example, it is my opinion that cost is the real reason why the Department of Health is using the excuse "until screening and treatment techniques are sufficiently well developed" as a moral smokescreen to justify why it will not implement a national screening programme for prostate cancer.

Also, how can a nation ranked 19th out of 22 countries in Europe for cancer survival beyond 5 years decide through its UK National Screening Committee (NSC) to delay any recommendation on screening for approximately 18 months after the European study was completed (see chapter 14 that follows for supporting information)?

Chapter 13: Author's Personal Opinion

The answer to this question from the UK NSC was, quote: "The trials were done in Europe and America where current attitudes to and uptake of PSA testing are different, they had a variety of thresholds, methods of diagnosis and treatment which need to be understood in the UK context".

When asked why they didn't take part in the European study their answer was, quote: "The UK NSC is not a research body. It takes results from research and applies them in a policy context. The UK NSC does not have services that test and treat men with raised PSA so we could not enter the trial".

These answers indicate to me that the UK NSC is there for "appearances only".

Another example that proves the Department of Health has no intention of introducing national screening for prostate cancer is the well recognised success of national screening for cervical cancer and breast cancer in women as can be seen from Graph 3 and Graph 4 respectively on the following page.

From Graph 3, deaths from cervical cancer have decreased dramatically since national screening started in 1967 to less than 1,000 deaths a year.

From Graph 4, breast cancer deaths were increasing and then dramatically started to drop after screening commenced in 1989.

Chapter 13: Author's Personal Opinion

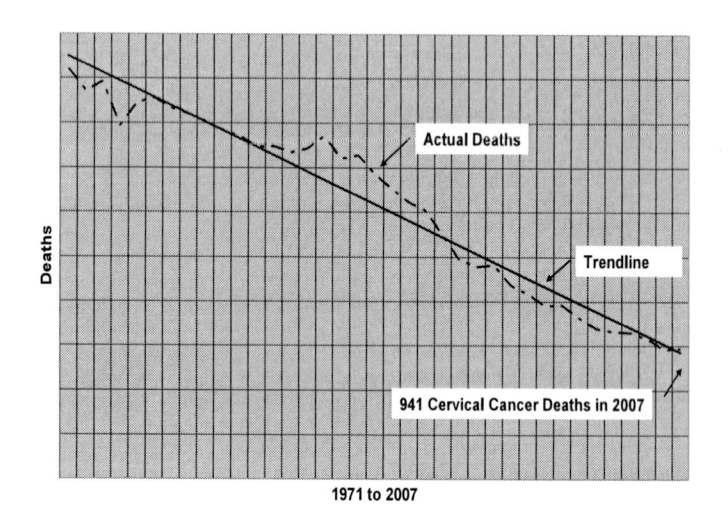

Graph 3: Cervical Cancer Deaths 1971 to 2007

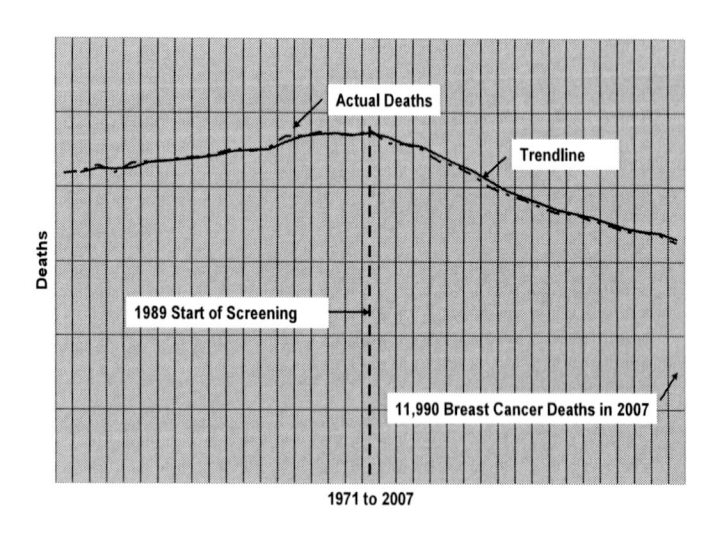

Graph 4: Breast Cancer Deaths 1971 to 2007

Chapter 13: Author's Personal Opinion

These two charts clearly indicate to me, and hopefully to you, that a significant number of men's lives will be saved by the introduction of national screening for prostate cancer.

Also, media reports recently indicated that 91.9% of men with prostate cancer in the USA were still alive after 5 years compared with only 51.1% in Britain. As the USA has national screening and Britain does not, this again is another clear indication of the benefit of national screening. For example, applying the same survival rate to the UK as the USA would save approximately 4,500 men's lives each year.

Why should male cancers behave differently than female cancers? And why should women have the privilege of national screening when men cannot?

Surely, this is discrimination as well as being contrary to human rights?

Another interesting point mentioned in the news recently is that many women are having mastectomies unnecessarily as some of the tumours being removed are believed to be very slow growing and therefore not life threatening.

Also, it has been found that some women with abnormal cervical smear results are being treated unnecessarily as the body can clear up these abnormalities itself without intervention. This unnecessary treatment can later cause complications in pregnancy,

Chapter 13: Author's Personal Opinion

These two recent findings are similar to the "pussycat" type of prostate cancer, which is also not life threatening.

If this recent news on breast cancer and cervical cancer is true does this mean that the department of Health will stop national screening for both these cancers?

Based on pure logic and common sense it is patently obvious that "Awareness" and lack of "Screening" are the main causes of "Late Diagnosis", the main reason why the UK was ranked 19th out of 22 countries for 5 year cancer survival rates in Europe.

Interestingly, only the Eastern European countries of Poland, The Czech Republic and Slovenia were ranked lower than the UK. In other words, the UK was at the bottom of the table as far as Western European Countries were concerned. What happened to the "Great" in Great Britain? And, most importantly, what has happened to the NHS, the supposedly envy of the world?

As mentioned previously, the UK NSC is concerned about the effectiveness of PSA testing to reliably identify prostate cancer and most importantly to identify whether the cancer is a "pussycat" or the aggressive life threatening "tiger" kind.

Chapter 13: Author's Personal Opinion

In the USA (the leaders in this area) a research team at Michigan University has found a marker, sarcosine, which can be detected in men's urine and discriminate between "tigers" and "pussycats".

It would seem sensible to me for the UK to explore the suitability of this marker to replace the PSA test. However, I suspect that because it is "Not Invented Here" it will probably be ignored

Going back to my earlier comment about the moral smokescreen excuse, the UK NSC are making particular reference to the 48 men that need to be treated to save one man's life, according to the European Randomised study.

What the UK NSC fails to highlight is that complications are being continually reduced as new treatment techniques are being developed and robotics are being used to minimise human error.

From a number of sources, complications are approximately 20%, which means for every man's life saved less than 10 men will experience complications. Surely, no matter how unpleasant these complications are, one man's life must be worth more than 10 men with complications?

In my opinion, the UK NSC is a typical public sector committee that suffers from the disease "paralysis through analysis" a very common disease in committees formed by the Government when they want to slow down or stop something from happening.

Chapter 13: Author's Personal Opinion

Another observation is that the National Awareness and Early Diagnosis Initiative (NAEDI) have no plans in the foreseeable future to produce a Cancer Awareness Measure (CAM) specifically for prostate cancer.

It seems the reason why a CAM is not being produced is that prostate camcer charities and/or the Government are not willing to fund the campaign.

To me, this means there is no desire in the "establishment" to prove beyond doubt that the reason why men are dying unnecessarily and living less than they should is lack of awareness of the symptoms and risks of prostate cancer.

As you can see I blame the Government for my predicament. At the beginning of this chapter I mentioned that some of you might think it is my fault for not being aware and taking control of my own health.

My defence in response to this is that I was under the illusion (not any more) that the NHS looks after the nation's health.

Why? Because of all the screening programmes already in place and the significant number of public information media broadcasts covering the need to stop smoking, minimise alcohol intake, stop taking drugs, lose weight, exercise, eat a healthy diet, etc.

Chapter 13: Author's Personal Opinion

Even thought I could continue with more examples, I feel "enough is enough" and it is now time for the various Prostate Cancer Support Organisations, the Prostate Cancer Support Federation and associated Charities, to "up their game", "get off the fence" and start actively lobbying the Government for change.

In addition, the real "Stakeholders" (men with prostate cancer and those affected or likely to be affected by prostate cancer) need to become more proactive to increase awareness of the symptoms and risks of prostate cancer for the benefit of all men and not just the privileged and fortunate few.

Sincere Regards

Doug Gray

Important:

Even though the Author is undoubtedly very, very annoyed and blames the Government for his predicament, he admires, respects and acknowledges the care and professionalism of the health professionals he has experienced, and continues to experience, with regard to his prostate cancer treatment and care.

The Author also admires, respects and acknowledges the efforts of many organisations and individuals who are very active, such as Prostate Cancer Support Organisations, the Prostate Cancer Support Federation, the Graham Fulford Charity, the Prostate Cancer Charity and individuals such as Andy Ripley, ex England Rugby International, who are very active in making men more aware of the symptoms and risks of prostate cancer.

Chapter 14

Facts and Supporting Information

Facts

- 35,000 men are diagnosed with prostate cancer every year in the UK.
- 10,000 men die each year of prostate cancer in the UK.
- Like cervical and breast cancer in women the earlier prostate cancer is diagnosed the greater the probability of a cure.
- Like cervical and breast cancer in women the later prostate cancer is diagnosed the more life threatening and incurable the cancer becomes.
- About a third of prostate cancers are diagnosed at an advanced stage when they are incurable thus resulting in eventual death from the disease.
- The reason why the UK was recently ranked only 19th out of 22 countries in Europe for cancer survival beyond 5 years is late diagnosis.
- The main cause of late diagnosis of prostate cancer in the UK is lack of awareness of the symptoms and risks of the disease.
- The 5 year survival rate for prostate cancer in the USA is 91.9% compared with only 51.1% in Britain.
- The USA has a national screening programme for prostate cancer but the UK does not.
- A recent *"European Randomised Study of Screening for Prostate Cancer"* concluded that around 20% of lives can be saved each year by national (Population) screening.

Chapter 14: Facts and Supporting Information

- The UK Department of Health will not implement a national prostate cancer screening programme until screening and treatment techniques are sufficiently well developed.

Supporting Information
- A national screening programme for prostate cancer will:
    - Save lives and increase life expectancy
    - Initially stretch the resources of the NHS
    - Cost the Government a significant amount of money
    - Increase the number of complications caused by the current treatment procedures available
- A national awareness campaign by the department of health, using appropriate medias, such as public information broadcasts on national TV and Radio, bulletins in the national press, posters in Doctors Surgeries, etc., will also:
    - Save lives and increase life expectancy
    - Cost the Government some money
    - Increase the number of men requesting tests for prostate cancer
    - Increase the number of complications caused by the current treatment procedures available
- On 18 March 2009, the UK National Screening Committee (NSC) was asked by Ministers to review its existing advice not to routinely screen for prostate cancer, following the publication of the European. Randomised Study of Screening for Prostate Cancer.
- The UK NSC formally reviewed this request at its meeting on 23rd June 2009, noting the European Randomised Study and new data from The Prostate, Lung, Colorectal and Ovarian Cancer Screening Trial in the United States.

Chapter 14: Facts and Supporting Information

- At the 23rd June meeting, the UK NSC agreed that the Sheffield School of Health And Related Research (ScHARR) should be commissioned to produce an independent academic analysis of the new trial data.
- This Sheffield School of Health And Related Research analysis is due to be completed in Spring 2010.
- Following the Sheffield School of Health And Related Research a stakeholder consultation will take place.
- After the consultation the UK NSC's updated advice will be formally published.
- The ProtecT Study (Prostate testing for cancer and Treatment) aims to evaluate treatments for localised prostate cancer and the outcome of each of the treatments. The study was open for recruitment from 2001-2008, but is not expected to deliver its findings until 2013.
- The National Awareness and Early Diagnosis Initiative (NAEDI) have no plans to develop a Cancer Awareness Measure (CAM) for prostate cancer in the foreseeable future.

Chapter 15

Support Organisations

The Prostate Cancer Charity www.prostate-cancer.org.uk
Tele: 0800 074 8383

Chestnut Appeal Charity: www.chestnutappeal.org.uk
Tele: 01752 792736

Prostate Cancer Support Federation
www.prostatecancerfederation.org.uk
Tele: 0845 601 0766

Prostate UK www.prostateuk.org
Tele: 020 8877 5840

Prostate Link UK www.prostate-link.org.uk

Cancer Research UK www.cancerresearchuk.org
Tele: 0808 800 4040

Cancerbackup www.cancerbackup.org.uk/Home
Tele: 0808 800 1234

Epilogue

At the time of publishing this book the Author, Doug Gray, has experienced rising PSA levels during the months of May, June, July, August and September 2009. During this period his testosterone levels remained low indicating that his hormone treatment was suppressing testosterone from the testes as intended.

Unfortunately, rising PSA and low testosterone levels meant that the cancer cells were very aggressive and had adapted themselves to feed on other male hormones. This being the case he started a treatment of daily tablets in September 2009 to provide total androgen (male hormones) blockade to slow down cancer growth.

Even though there are still a number of treatment options available, after the cancer cells mutate again to find something else to feed on, this is not a good sign as the first stage of hormone treatment can usually last a few years.

This said, the Author will continue to follow his strict dairy free and high antioxidant diet in the hope of delaying departure sufficiently long enough to make some headway in helping to increase the awareness of the symptoms and risks of prostate cancer.

About the Author

Doug Gray was diagnosed in early February 2009 at the age of 62 with advanced prostate cancer. As a consequence his priorities changed and he decided to actively campaign for the Greater Awareness of the Symptoms and Risks of Prostate Cancer.

To help communicate his awareness message, he has invested in his own web site www.loveyourprostate.co.uk on which he tells his story and provides some useful information on prostate cancer. He has also written and published this book to help the campaign.

Within a few months of being diagnosed, he became a media talker for the Prostate Cancer Charity and spoke at their launch of the "Hampered by Hormones" campaign at the House of Commons. He is also one of the three men filmed in the short video used to promote the "Hampered by Hormones" campaign.

At the time of writing this book he has been on BBC TV Spotlight in the South West, been interviewed live on BBC Radio Devon and BBC Radio Cornwall and featured in various local newspapers.

Doug also took the initiative to form a patient led Steering Group from like minded individuals of the Derriford Prostate Support Group with the main goal of providing greater awareness of the symptoms and risks of prostate cancer.

Glossary

CAM	Cancer Awareness Measure
DRE	Digital Rectum Examination
FDA	Food and Drug Administration (USA)
HDR	High Dose Rate
LDR	Low Dose Rate
NAEDI	National Awareness and Early Diagnosis Initiative
ProtecT	**Pro**state **te**sting for **c**ancer and **T**reatment
PSA	Prostate Specific Antigen
ScHARR	Sheffield School of Health And Related Research
UK NSC	UK National Screening Committee

Information Sources

Cancer Research UK www.cancerresearchuk.org

Cancer Research www.cancerresearchuk.org

Chestnut Appeal Charity www.chestnutappeal.org.uk

NAEDI www.info.cancerresearchuk.org

National Statistics www.statistics.gov.uk

Office of National Statistics www.ons.gov.uk

Prostate Cancer Support Federation
www.prostatecancerfederation.org.uk

Prostate UK www.prostateuk.org

ProtecT Study www.epi.bris.ac.uk

Prostate Cancer Charity www.prostate-cancer.org.uk

UK Department of Health www.dh.gov.uk

UK National Screening Committee www.screening.nhs.uk

Daily Mail Newspaper

Prostate Cancer, a Book by Professor Jane Plant
www.janeplant.com